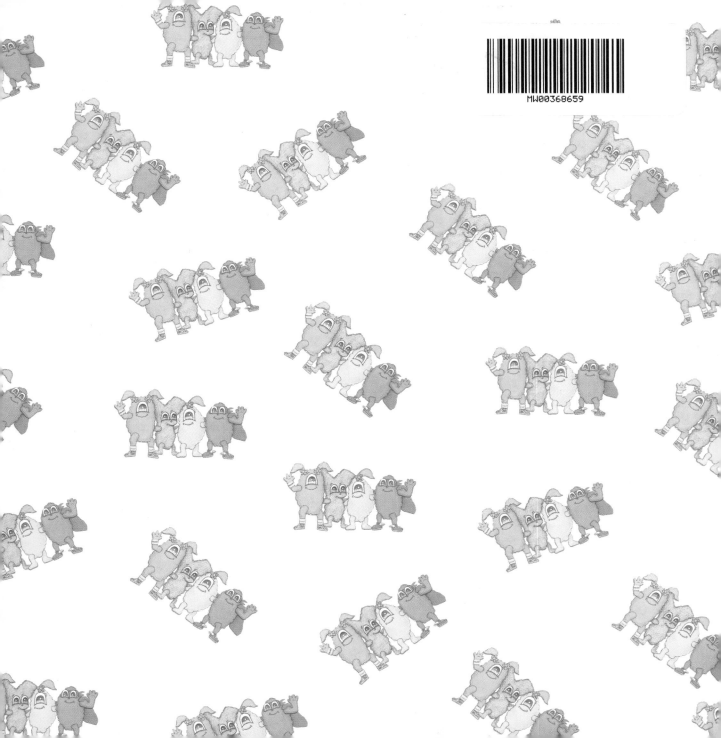

Buddies In My Belly: a story about probiotics

By Sarah Morgan + Henry Bell

For information contact
Buddies In My Belly
9185 E Kenyon Ave Suite 195
Denver, CO 80237
WWW.BUDDIESINMYBELLY.COM

Illustrated by Henry Bell
Proudly printed in the United States of America by Walsworth Publishing, Marceline, MO

ISBN 978-1-5323-5106-8

Let's Meet the Buddies

Probiotics are friendly bacteria that live in your body and help you stay healthy. They can help support the health of your digestive tract, immune system, brain, heart, lungs and even the absorption of nutrients and excretion of waste. Did you know that 2-4 pounds of your body weight is from the Buddies In Your Belly?

Lactie

Lactobacillus has been shown to help with the breakdown of food, including gluten and lactose. Lactobacillus can also help improve energy and mood through the production of the neurotransmitter, acetylcholine.

Biffie

Bifidobacterium is important for mood, sleep and focus due to its ability to make the calming neurotransmitter, GABA. Bifidobacterium also helps move food through the digestive tract to minimize gas, bloating and constipation.

Strepie

Streptococcus strains are important for ear, nose and throat health. Having the right forms of streptococcus in the mouth may help inhibit cavities and strep throat infections.

Ba-Silly

Bacillus is a spore-forming bacteria that has been shown to boost the immune system and strengthen DNA. Bacillus can also help with memory, focus and energy through the production of neurotransmitters, dopamine and norepinephrine.

For more information about Buddies In My Belly™ and our products, please visit:

WWW.BUDDIESINMYBELLY.COM

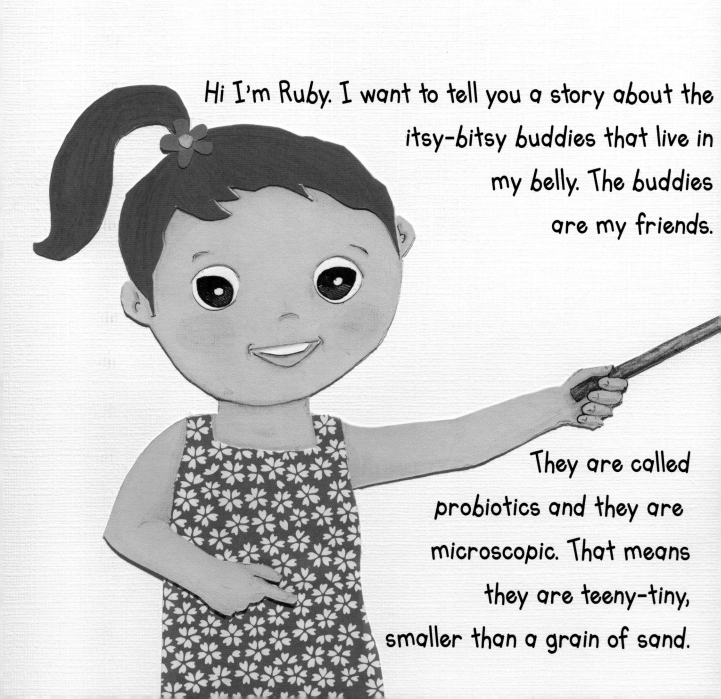

Hi I'm Ruby. I want to tell you a story about the itsy-bitsy buddies that live in my belly. The buddies are my friends.

They are called probiotics and they are microscopic. That means they are teeny-tiny, smaller than a grain of sand.

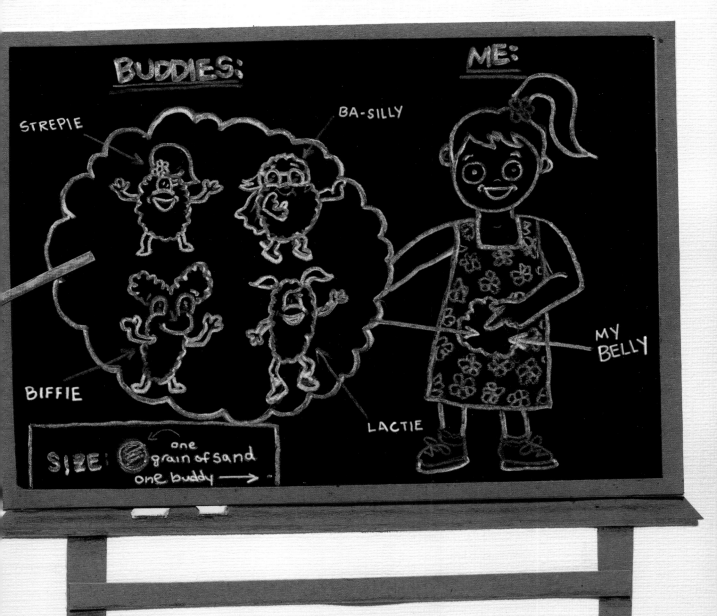

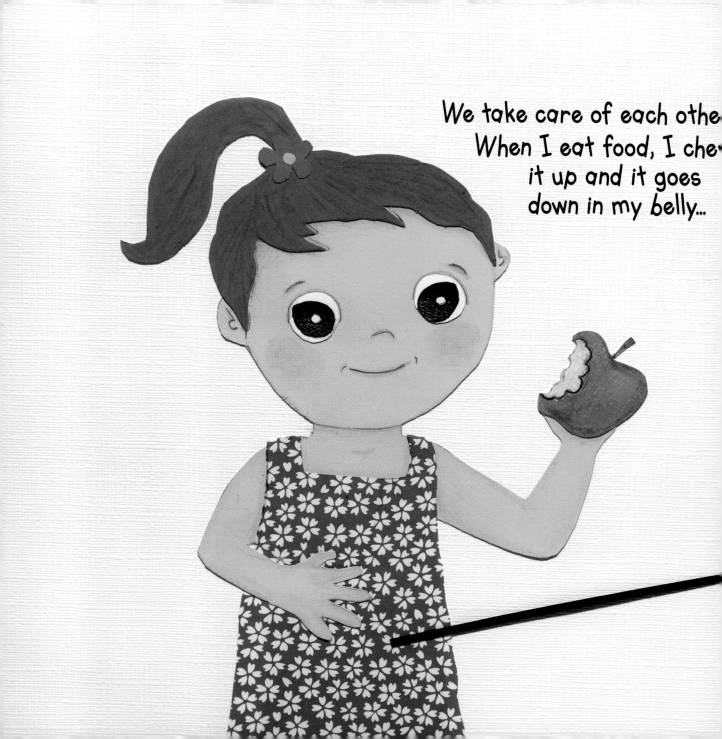

We take care of each othe
When I eat food, I che
it up and it goes
down in my belly...

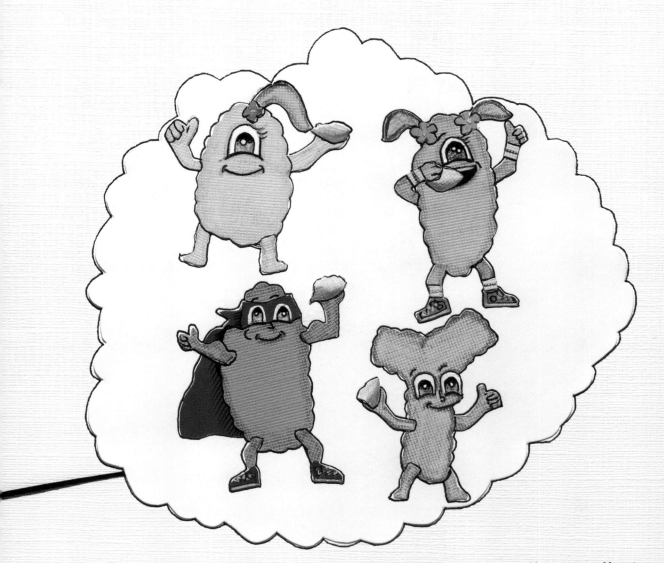

And the buddies keep chewing the food and pull out all the
vitamins and minerals and nutrients to keep me healthy.

This is Lactie. She is my favorite buddy for helping me digest my food.

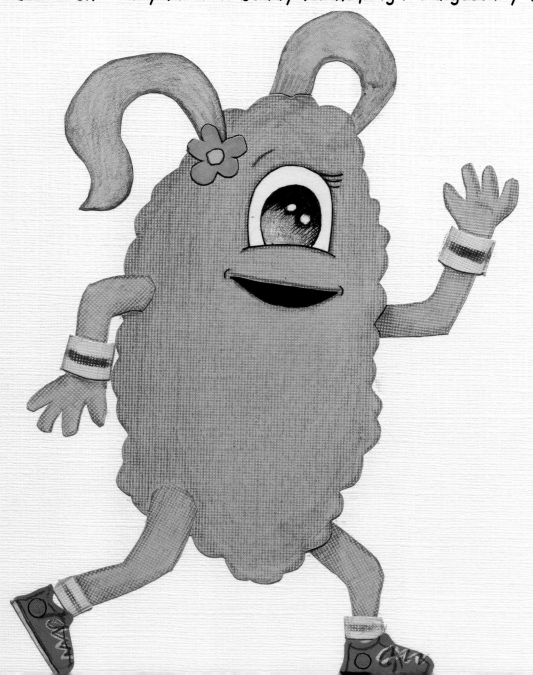

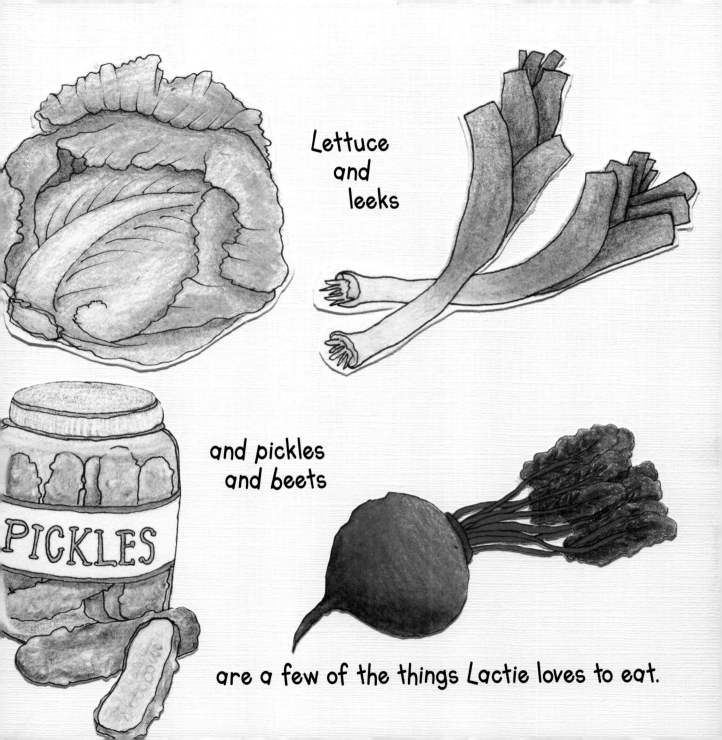

Lettuce
and
leeks

and pickles
and beets

PICKLES

are a few of the things Lactie loves to eat.

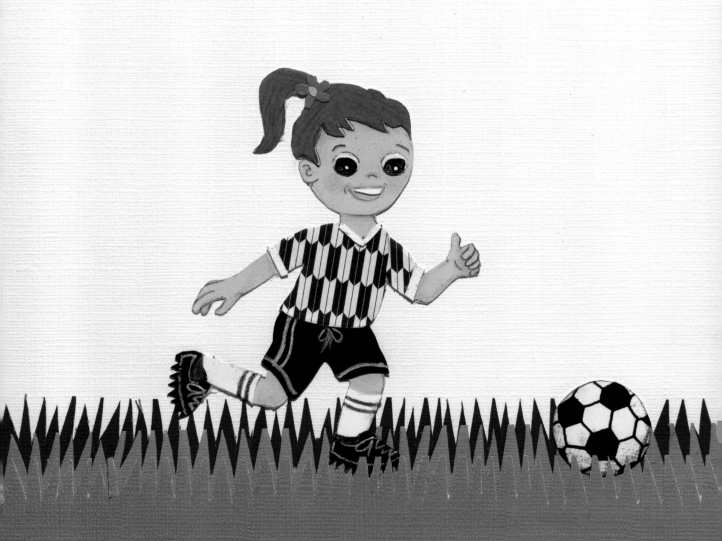

When I feed Lactie her favorite foods, she gives me energy and keeps me in a good mood.

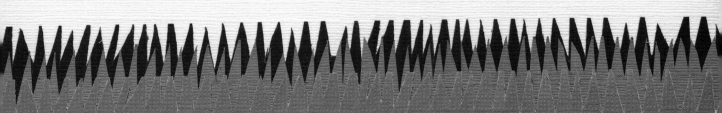

This is Biffie. He is my favorite buddy to help me go poop.

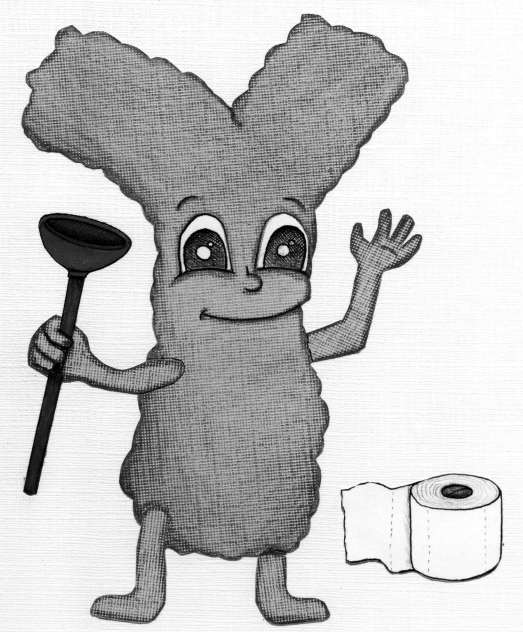

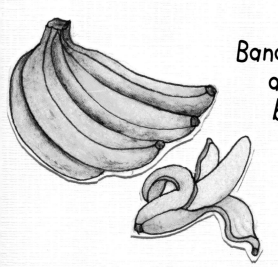

Bananas
and
broccoli

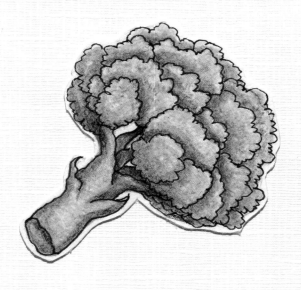

and berries
and beans

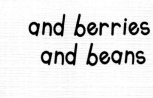

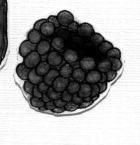

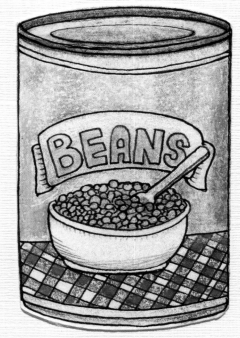

are a few of Biffie's favorite things.

When I feed Biffie his favorite food, he helps me make a perfect poop.

Sometimes he even makes me toot...

Awww Biffie!

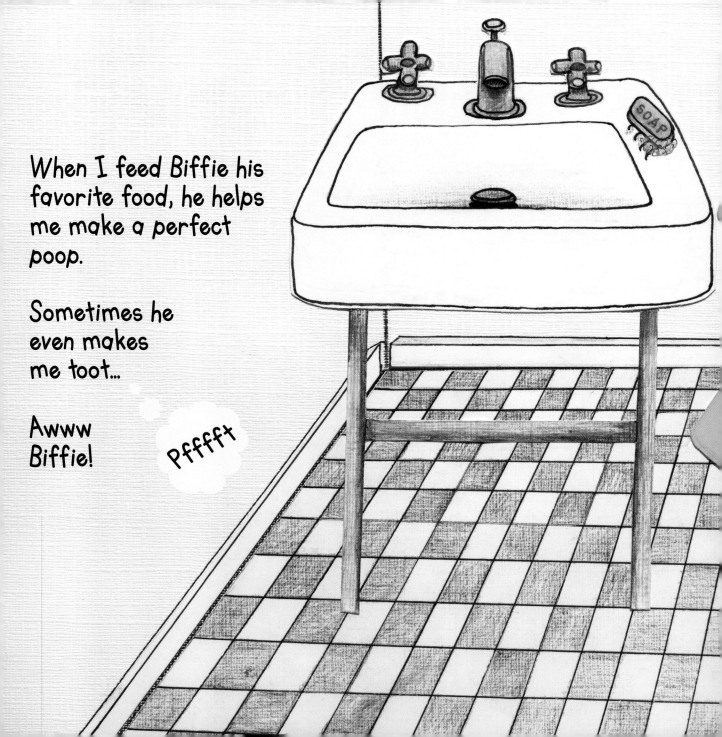

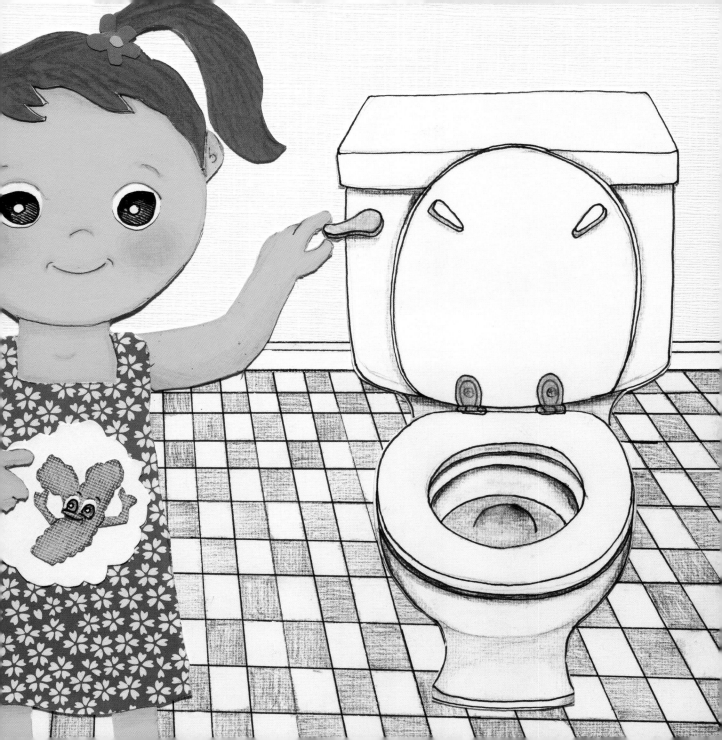

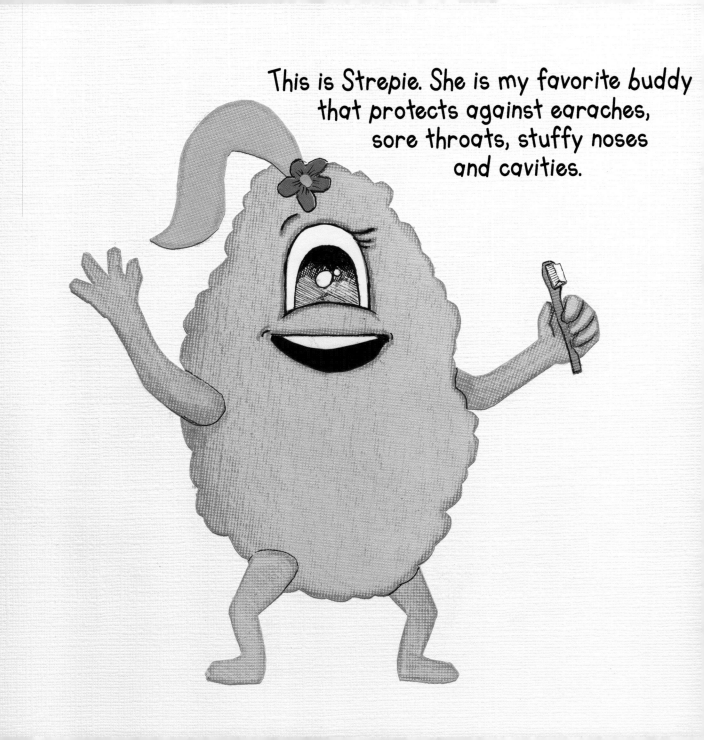

This is Strepie. She is my favorite buddy that protects against earaches, sore throats, stuffy noses and cavities.

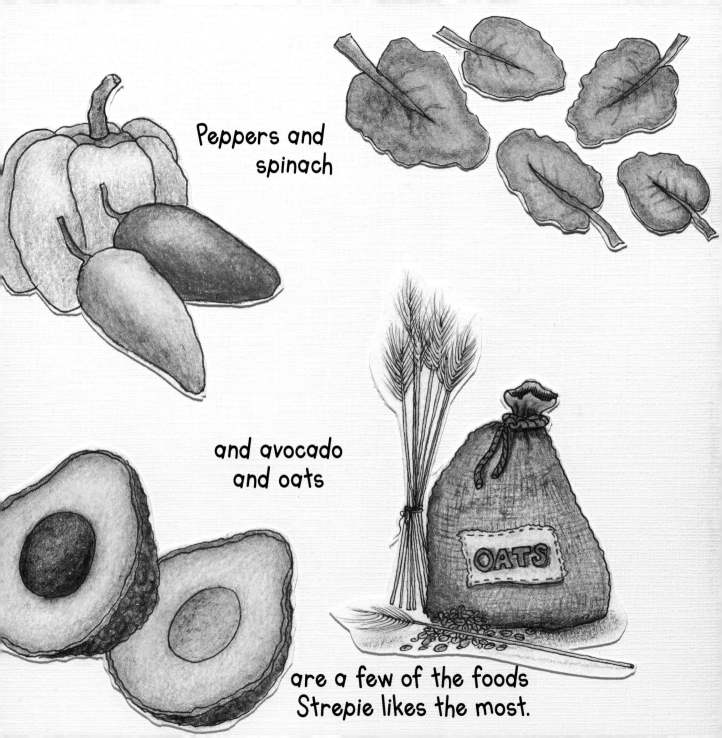

Peppers and spinach

and avocado and oats

are a few of the foods Strepie likes the most.

When I feed Strepie her favorite foods, she
is the key crusader in fighting off my ear,
nose and throat foreign invaders.

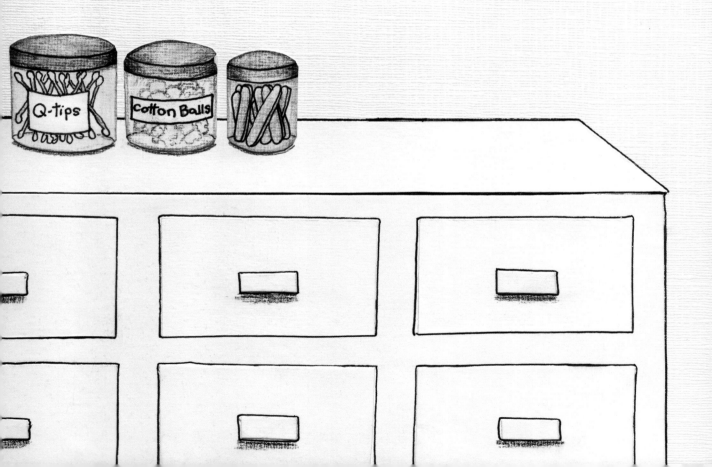

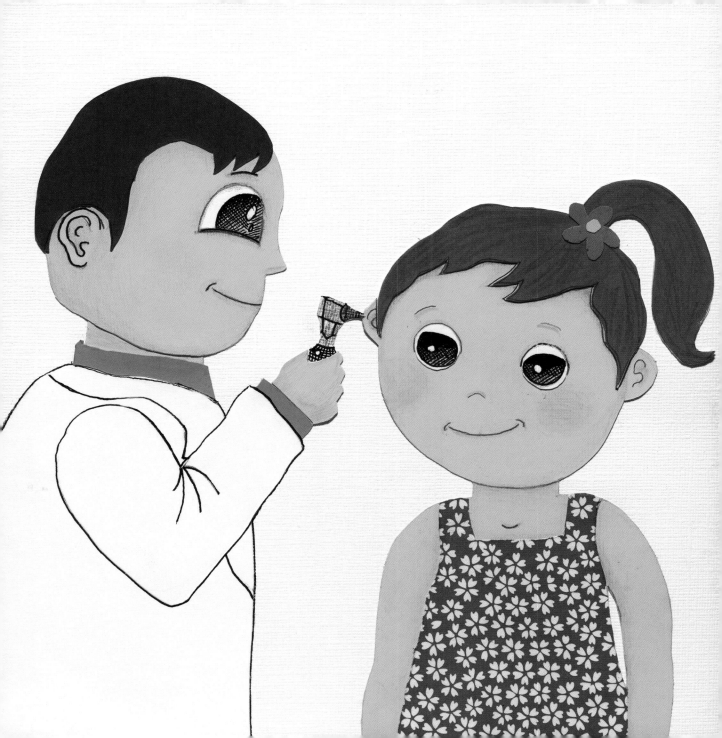

This is Ba-silly. He is my favorite buddy for protecting me against colds.

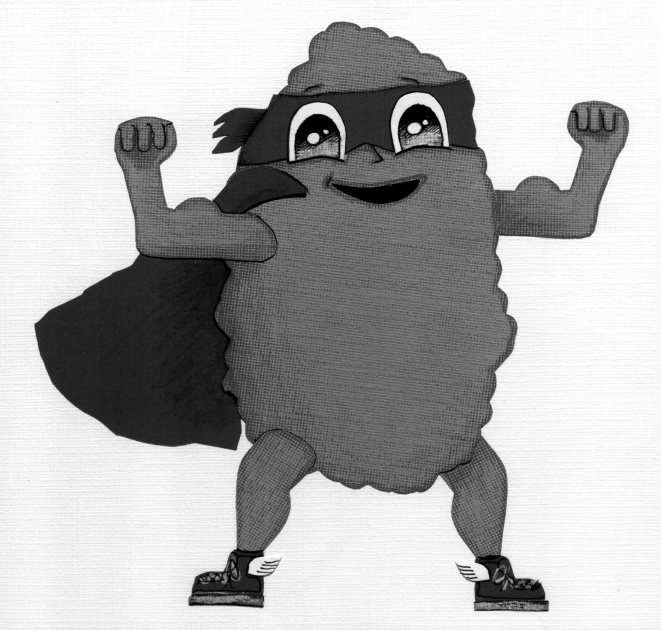

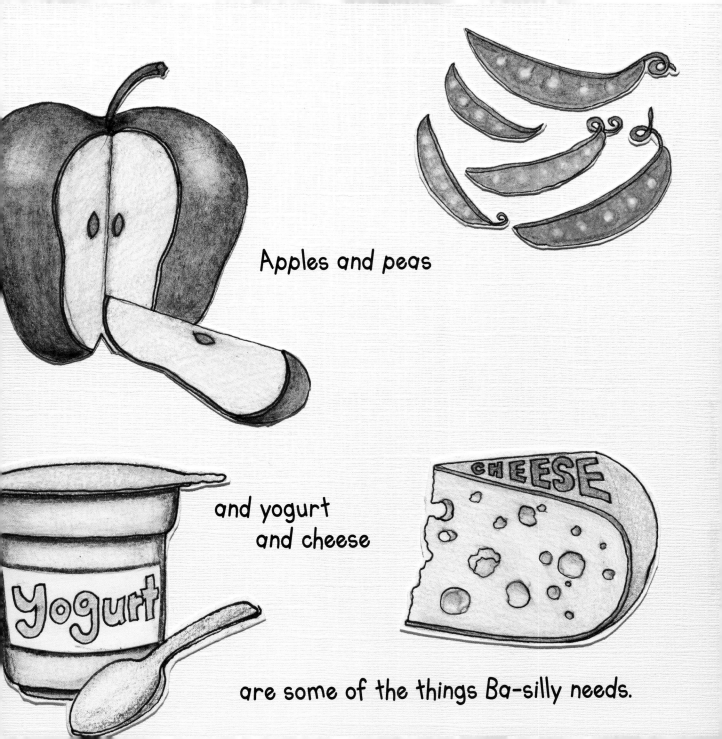

Apples and peas

and yogurt
and cheese

are some of the things Ba-silly needs.

When Ba-silly eats his favorite food, he gets in a superhero mood. Bad germs don't stand a chance against Ba-Silly's superhero stance. Hi-Yah!

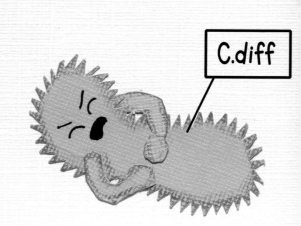

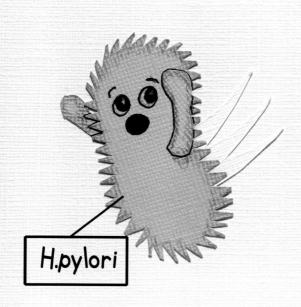

H.pylori

C.diff

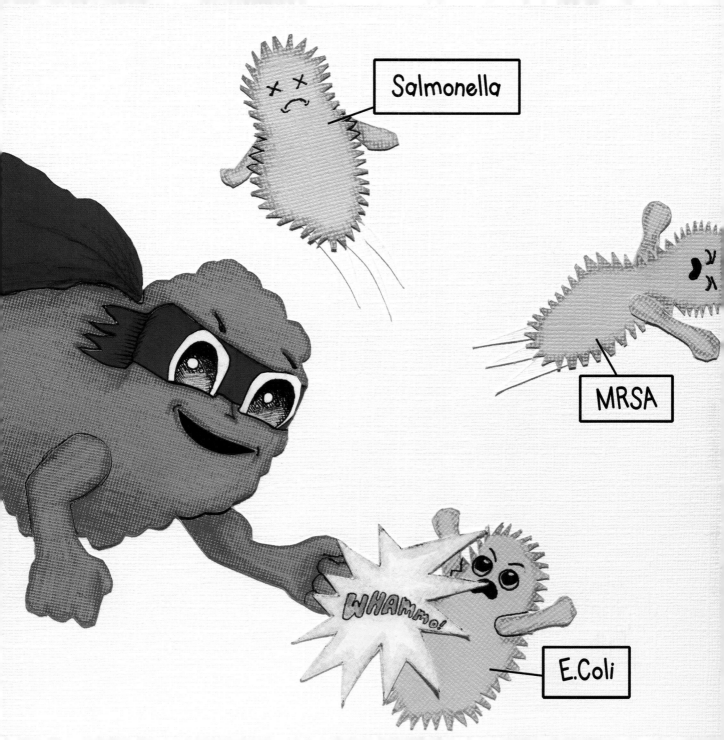

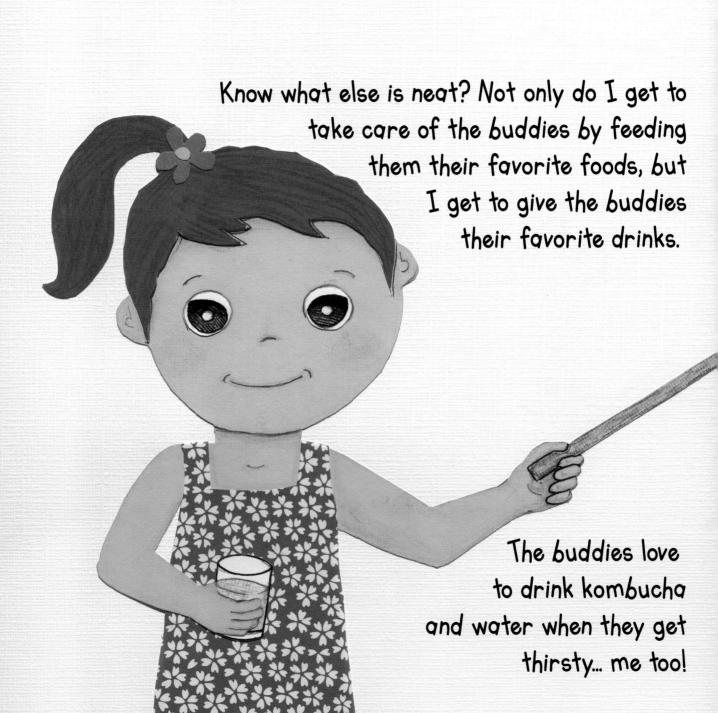

Know what else is neat? Not only do I get to take care of the buddies by feeding them their favorite foods, but I get to give the buddies their favorite drinks.

The buddies love to drink kombucha and water when they get thirsty... me too!

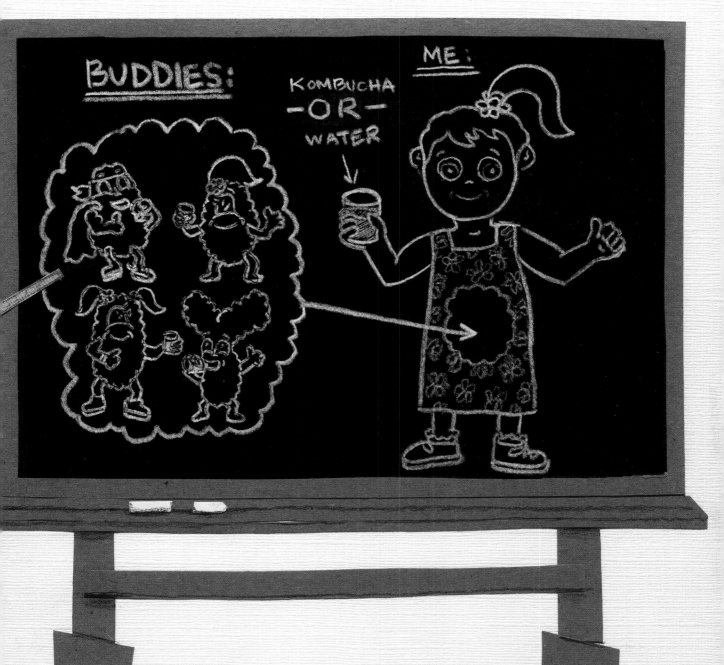

If I eat too much candy and cookies and ice cream...

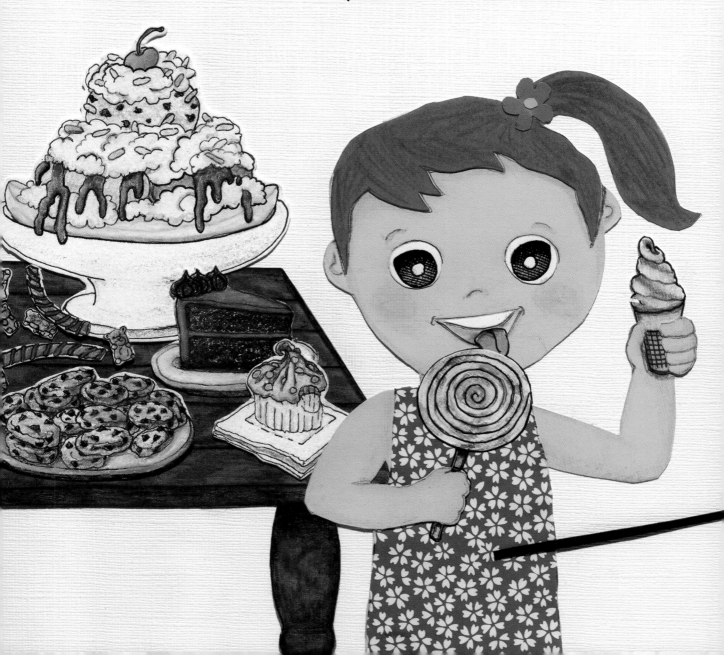

The buddies get sick. And when the buddies are sick they can't take care of me.

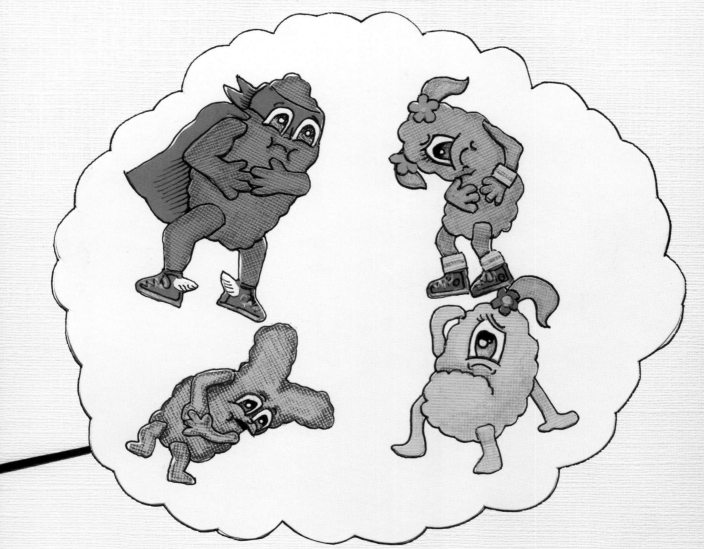

When I feed the buddies and take care of them,

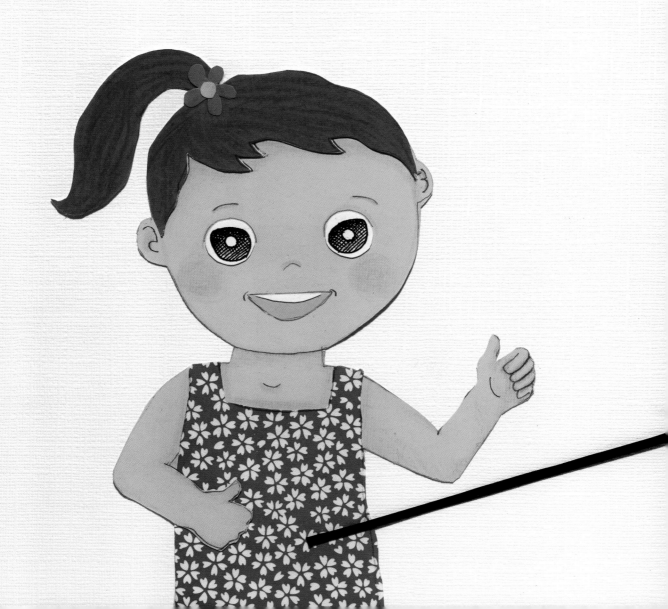

we all work together to *be happy* and healthy.

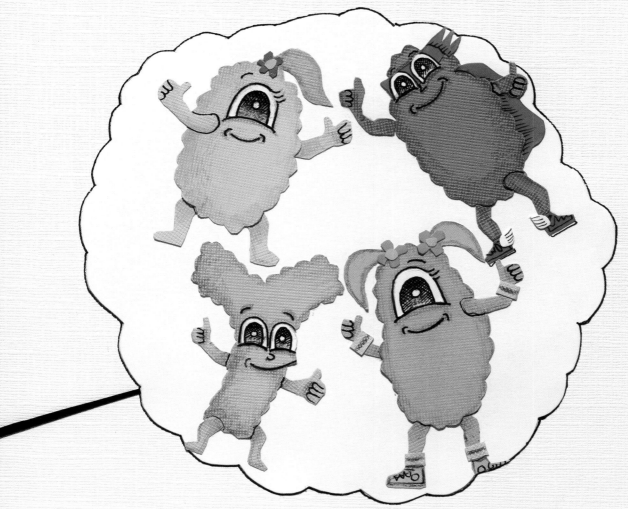

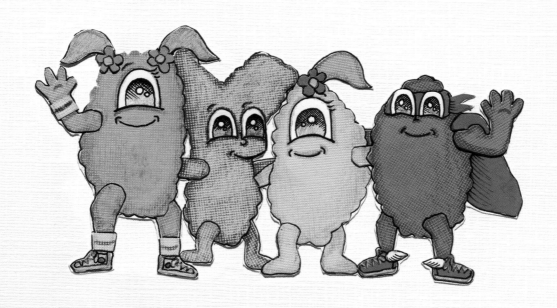

Now it's your turn to take care
of the *buddies* in your *belly.*

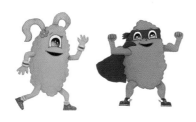 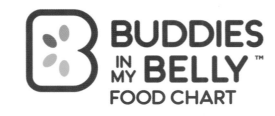 **BUDDIES IN MY BELLY™ FOOD CHART**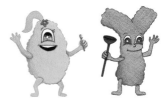

Red

			Sun	Mon	Tue	Wed	Thu	Fri	Sat
Apples	Grapes	Strawberries	★	★	★	★	★	★	★
Kidney beans	Plums	Tomatoes							
Beets	Potatoes	Watermelon	★	★	★	★	★	★	★
Bell peppers	Pomegranate								
Cherries	Raspberries								

Orange

			Sun	Mon	Tue	Wed	Thu	Fri	Sat
Apricot	Mango	Butternut squash	★	★	★	★	★	★	★
Bell peppers	Nectarine	Sweet potatoes							
Cantaloupe	Orange		★	★	★	★	★	★	★
Carrots	Pumpkin								

Yellow

			Sun	Mon	Tue	Wed	Thu	Fri	Sat
Banana	Corn	Pear	★	★	★	★	★	★	★
Bell peppers	Lemon	Pineapple	★	★	★	★	★	★	★

Green

			Sun	Mon	Tue	Wed	Thu	Fri	Sat
Apples	Celery	Lettuce	★	★	★	★	★	★	★
Asparagus	Cucumbers	Melon							
Avocado	Edamame	Olives	★	★	★	★	★	★	★
Bell peppers	Green beans	Peas							
Brussels sprouts	Kale	Pickles							
Broccoli	Lime	Spinach							
Cabbage	Leeks	Swiss chard							

Blue/Purple

			Sun	Mon	Tue	Wed	Thu	Fri	Sat
Blueberries	Eggplant	Potatoes	★	★	★	★	★	★	★
Blackberries	Figs	Raisins							
Cabbage	Grapes	Black/purple rice	★	★	★	★	★	★	★
Carrots	Plums								

White/Tan

			Sun	Mon	Tue	Wed	Thu	Fri	Sat
Applesauce	Legumes -	Quinoa	★	★	★	★	★	★	★
Bean dip	chickpeas,	Sauerkraut							
Brown rice	lentils, etc	Seeds	★	★	★	★	★	★	★
Coconut	Nuts								
Garlic	Oats								

*Aim for 1-2 servings of each color category per day

Tear off and put me on the fridge.

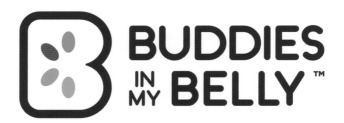

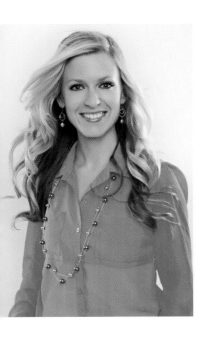

Sarah Morgan, The Gene Queen, is known for her innovative ideas that connect science to everyday life in a way that impacts thousands. Albert Einstein's quote, "If you can't explain it simply, you don't understand it well enough" has inspired Sarah to write and communicate in such a way that a 4-year old and a 40-year old will understand.

Sarah has a clinical practice in Denver, Colorado, that focuses on using food and nutrients to optimize gene expression and help individuals with complex health issues. Sarah is married to her best friend and champion, Matt, and finds her inspiration from her daughter, Madison.

Sarah earned her Bachelor's degree in Biology and Chemistry from the University of Wisconsin – Eau Claire. She holds a Masters of Science in Functional Nutrition from the University of Bridgeport. Sarah has worked in the health and nutrition field for the past 12 years helping individuals, communities and corporations achieve their health and wellness goals.

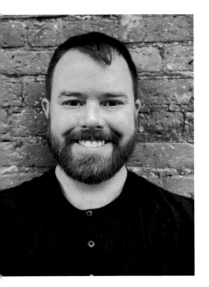

Henry Daniel Bell is a professional artist/illustrator born and raised in Denver, Colorado. With a Bachelor of the Arts degree from Southern Methodist University and over 30 years of artistic expression under his belt—Henry has committed his life to the arts. Henry is an avid rock climber, loves restoring classic cars and motorcycles and has traveled extensively studying art around the world.

Henry married his beautiful wife, Heather, in 2011. Henry and Heather and their two dogs, Mason and Ryu, live part time in Maui, Hawaii and part time in Denver, Colorado. Henry is a proud uncle to nine incredible kiddos and took much of his inspiration for this book from his nieces and nephews. He hopes that this book will positively influence children to be more conscious about what they eat and the role the microbiome plays in their overall health. Eat-well, live-long and prosper!

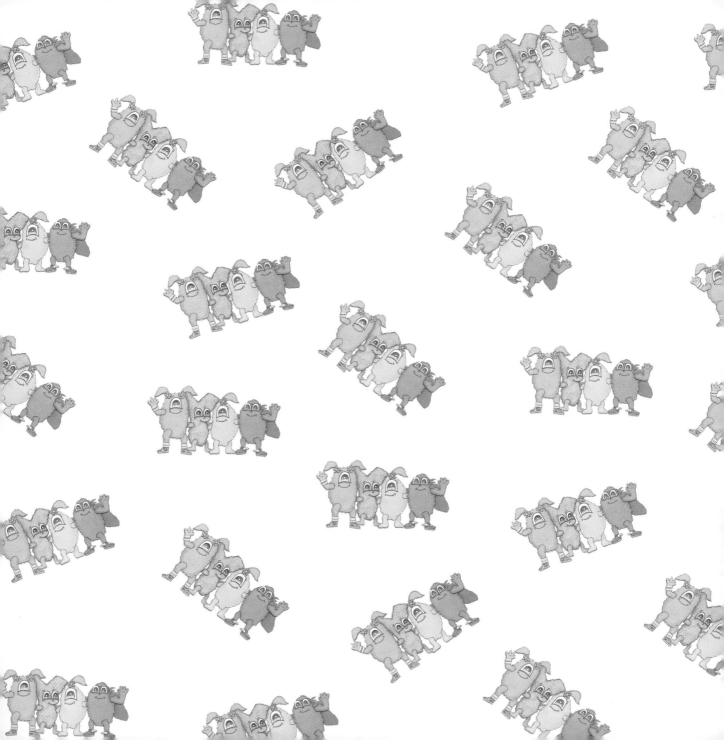

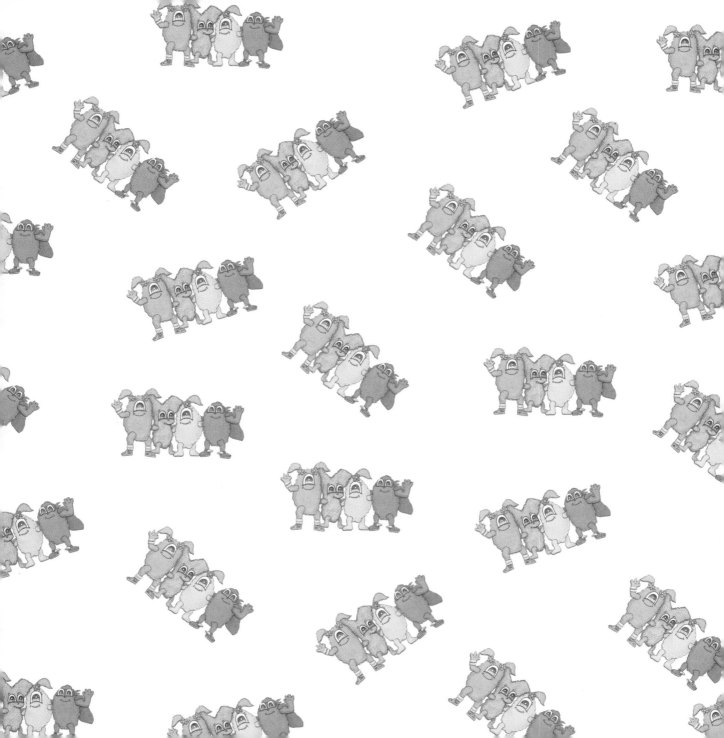

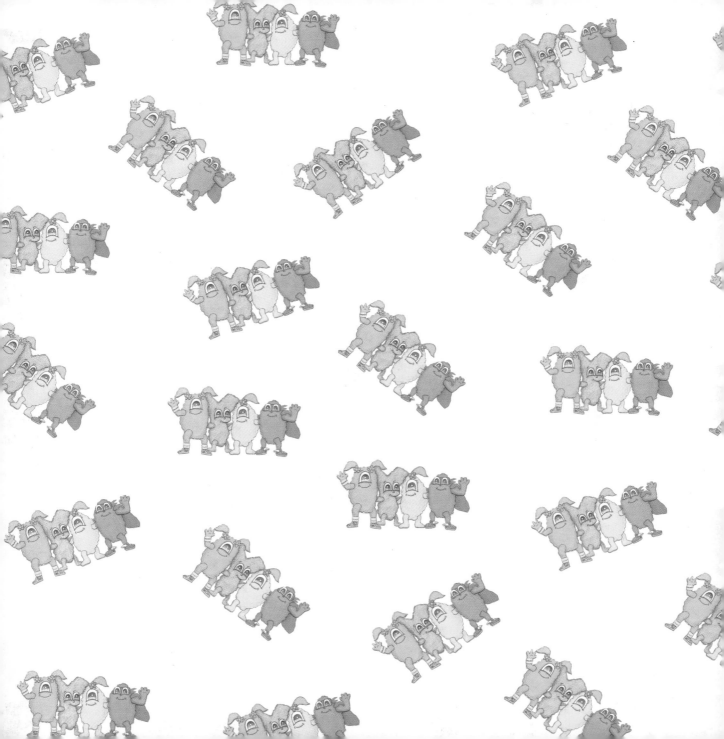